HOW TO LOSE BELLY FAT

ANTHONY EKANEM

Copyright © Anthony Ekanem
All Rights Reserved.

This book has been self-published with all reasonable efforts taken to make the material error-free by the author. No part of this book shall be used, reproduced in any manner whatsoever without written permission from the author, except in the case of brief quotations embodied in critical articles and reviews.

The Author of this book is solely responsible and liable for its content including but not limited to the views, representations, descriptions, statements, information, opinions and references ["Content"]. The Content of this book shall not constitute or be construed or deemed to reflect the opinion or expression of the Publisher or Editor. Neither the Publisher nor Editor endorse or approve the Content of this book or guarantee the reliability, accuracy or completeness of the Content published herein and do not make any representations or warranties of any kind, express or implied, including but not limited to the implied warranties of merchantability, fitness for a particular purpose. The Publisher and Editor shall not be liable whatsoever for any errors, omissions, whether such errors or omissions result from negligence, accident, or any other cause or claims for loss or damages of any kind, including without limitation, indirect or consequential loss or damage arising out of use, inability to use, or about the reliability, accuracy or sufficiency of the information contained in this book.

Made with ♥ on the Notion Press Platform
www.notionpress.com

Contents

Preface v

1. What Is Belly Fat? 1

2. Benefits Of Losing Weight 3

3. Tips To Reduce Belly Fat 7

Conclusion 21

Preface

Abdominal obesity, also known as central obesity, is something that many people worldwide have problems with. Once they hit middle age, many people are plagued by those two dreaded words, belly fat. It can, however, also be a problem for children and teens.

People just look at it as a weight problem, but it can also be linked to cardiovascular disease, Alzheimer's disease, and many other metabolic and vascular diseases.

Though no one likes belly fat, too often, it is overlooked as just a symptom of age. It can, however, be a symptom of something more serious. It is not something you should just consider the price of getting older. It is something that should be taken seriously.

CHAPTER ONE

What is Belly Fat?

Usually, belly fat is subcutaneous fat, which is underneath the skin. If you have problems with abdominal fat, it may also be visceral fat. This is also known as organ fat which is packed between the internal organs. This is also known as the "pot belly" or the "beer belly." It is associated with type-2 diabetes, cardiovascular disease, and colorectal cancer.

In recent studies, scientists have come to realize that it is not really how much a person weighs – it is the amount of body fat that truly indicates obesity.

Throughout the 1980s and 90s, imaging techniques were developed that helped improve the understanding of how many health risks can be associated with the accumulation of body fat. These include tomography and magnetic resonance which help divide masses of tissue in the abdominal region.

For women, belly fat is more common after menopause. Sometimes, people just think this goes hand-in-hand with getting older, and don't realize the danger it can cause. While women feel like it is just something that makes them go up a size in their jeans, it does carry health risks.

Like fat in any other part of the body, it is determined by balancing the calories you take in with the energy you burn.

In other words, if you eat too much and burn too little, you will have excess fat. As you get older, your muscle mass reduces. Your fat, however, increases. When your muscle mass reduces, it also reduces the rate your body uses calories. This can make it even more difficult for people to maintain a weight that is healthy as they age.

Sometimes, you can have an increase in belly fat as you age without even gaining weight. In women, this can be due to a reduced level of estrogen. Research has shown that estrogen seems to influence where the fat is distributed in a woman's body. Regardless of the weight shown as normal on the BMI measurement charts, women with a large waistline have been known to carry the risk of premature death and often die earlier of cardiovascular disease.

Most women hate to even have an inch or so too much belly fat. How do you know, however, if the belly fat you carry is a health risk? Just measure it. Use a tape measure and place it around your bare stomach. You want it to be snug, but not cut into the skin. For women, if your measurement is over 35 inches, you'll be at a greater risk for health problems. For men, the measurement of concern is around 40 inches.

People who are plagued with belly fat often exercise and participate in healthy activities, yet they still retain that unwanted fat. It seems like the fat is immune to exercise. So how do you get rid of it? What is the magic combination that says "poof" to that extra poundage? It depends on your sex, age, and the number of pounds you want to lose, but there are many tips to help you reduce that unwanted belly fat.

CHAPTER TWO

Benefits of Losing Weight

Losing weight isn't always easy, and as a result, it can harm your self-esteem. It is, however, important for you to main a normal weight for more than cosmetic reasons. You need to maintain proper health for many health reasons. In a society like ours, where people put such importance on the way they look, feeling unattractive can lead to serious depression. While not all overweight people get depressed, some are, in fact, quite happy the way they are, and it can lead to serious emotional and mental problems in addition to other health problems.

It can be difficult to determine how much weight you need to lose to be healthy. You should realize, however, that you don't have to lose weight if you're not overweight. More important than weight, is the amount of fat content you have in your body and where that fat has accumulated. Sometimes, you have weight gain because you've started working out and developed muscles. Muscles are heavier than fat, so don't be shocked if all that exercise has reduced inches but increased weight. If this is the case, there's no problem at all and you don't have to worry about losing that weight.

While being too worried about our weight can be a problem too, knowing you're overweight and taking the steps to reduce that weight is important. There are many benefits to losing weight. Here are a few of them:

- Reduces your risk of long-term health problems that could shorten your life. These include health problems such as diabetes and cardiovascular disease. Usually, this is the main reason people find to lose weight.

- Feeling better, healthier, and having more energy. You'll be able to take the stairs or walk from the far end of the parking lot without losing your breath.

- Less pain in your joints. Problems such as osteoarthritis in your knees and pain and swelling in your ankles can greatly be reduced. Being overweight puts a strain on them that you will feel greatly reduced when you lose weight.

- Many times when you lose weight, especially if you're diabetic or have high blood pressure, your doctor will be able to take you off your medication. Not only will you be healthier and not take so much medication, but you'll also save a lot of money at the pharmacy counter.

- You'll feel better about yourself as you gradually join the people with smaller mid-sections. Your self-esteem will increase. You'll find yourself interacting with others in a whole new way.

- When you are eating out with co-worker you won't be overeating, so it could advance your career. Believe it or not, behaviour specialists have studied this, and they found that eating healthy gives you the impression of a person that is outcome driven. This is something supervisors look for. When they see it in you, they take a closer look at you as an employee. Don't be surprised if you've looked at a promotion you never thought you'd get.

- Save money — This is a given. If you eat less, naturally you won't be buying as much food when you eat out and when you eat at home. You'll save money all the way around. You could even put aside the extra money you normally spend on food. When your weight loss is complete, you could have enough money for a whole new wardrobe or a nice vacation to treat yourself. After all, you'll look great. You will have worked hard, so you deserve a treat.

- Keep your sex drive and be more satisfied sexually — This is especially true for men. There have been studies that show if a man is around 30 pounds overweight, he can have the testosterone levels of a man that is at least 10 years older. This reduces their sex drive. Other tests have also shown that people who are obese are much less satisfied with their sexual experiences. Sex is an important part of your life, especially for those in a relationship. You want to get the most out of it. Stay fit and you will.

- You can have more friends — Face it, overweight people can sometimes be outcasts. Sometimes, it's self-inflicted, but other times, people just stay away from the "fat" person. When you lose weight, you'll feel more like making friends. You'll be able to participate in more activities which will allow you to meet more people. You'll make friends from circles you didn't dream of before.

- Influence others — Sometimes, especially with spouses, one losing weight can be a positive influence on the other and cause them to lose weight as well. If your children are overweight as well, it could be a genetic issue. Influencing them to begin losing weight before it gets as "out of control" as it is for you can give them a head start on the genetic problem and like Barney says, "Nip it!"

CHAPTER THREE

Tips to Reduce Belly Fat

Fortunately, belly fat can be eliminated or reduced by the same means that other fat can. It just takes the right combination of diet and exercise. There are, however, other factors that can hinder weight loss and cause you to retain belly fat. Below are tips that can help you reduce that belly fat:

1. **Avoid stress** — Research has found that our bodies produce hormones in response to stress. One of these is cortisol. It will cause your body to look for high-calorie food because it thinks it used a lot of energy handling something stressful. It's kind of like tricking your body into thinking it's had a big workout, when in fact, it's done nothing but become anxious and upset. Years ago, eating that type of high-calorie food was fine when you were stressed because you used more energy every day working in the fields or on farms. Our ancestors remained thin during stressful times because of their hard work.

Now, many of us live more sedentary lives. We simply can't burn that type of fat intake any longer. When you're under a large amount of chronic stress, it tells your body to keep on making cortisol. It becomes a vicious cycle.

Gaining weight makes you even more stressed, so you produce more cortisol and eat more fattening foods.

You can reduce stress by doing several things. You can get more sleep. The average adult should get at least seven hours of sleep a night. You should keep things that are stressful away from the area you use for sleeping. Don't do work in bed if you can help it. That area should be for relaxation instead of work. Simply work at leaving your worries outside the bedroom door.

You should also set aside some time to relax each day. By closing your eyes, breathing deeply, and forgetting your worries for a brief period, even if it's only 15 minutes a day, you can help reduce stress. Exercise will also help by giving you an outlet for stress. Keeping your blood sugar level will also help.

2. **Tell friends/family that you're dieting** — By telling others that you're dieting, you have them to help keep you in check. Of course, you'll hear things like, "You're dieting aren't you" or "Are you supposed to be eating that," but it will help you stick to your diet. You'll also hear things like, "How much have you lost" or "You're looking so good." Those things can be very encouraging. Once you've made the proclamation that you're dieting, you'll feel like you have to prove you can do it, so you're more apt to stick with it and achieve success.

3. **Diet with a friend** — Having a "buddy" system when you diet is a great way to lose weight. You have someone to help keep you in check, but you also have someone you can eat out with that you won't have to explain you're dieting or someone that will be eating fattening foods in front of you. You can help and encourage each other along the way. You can celebrate each success you make as well as the success of your friends.

4. **Stop smoking and/or drinking** — People often say if they stop smoking they'll gain weight and use that as an excuse to keep smoking. That is all it is...an excuse! Both smoking and drinking will cause you to gain weight and keep stubborn belly fat. Find something else to do with the time you usually spend smoking. Take short walks, exercise, or do something else that is healthy and good for your body instead of smoking which you know is harmful to your body.

5. **Eat** — I know it may seem like a counterproductive measure, but it isn't. Eating is important when you're trying to reduce your weight, including trying to lose your stubborn belly fat. Breakfast is extremely important when you're dieting. Many people will skip breakfast to lose weight, but that's one of the worst things you can do. It has been proven that eating about an hour after you wake up can keep your insulin levels steadier and aid in keeping your weight steadier. You don't want to eat a whole pig and a dozen eggs, but eating a breakfast that is high in fibre and protein can boost your body's metabolism and help you burn fat. Foods like eggs, fresh fruits/vegetables, or peanut butter are better for you than the more sugary things such as breakfast cereals, pancakes, or pastries.

It is also better to eat four to five small meals a day than eat one or two large ones. This way you keep the signal to your body that is going to get fuel. If you don't, or if you eat at irregular times and in irregular amounts, your body won't know it is going to constantly get fuel. It thinks it has to store that fat for future energy use. Usually, where does it store it...right around the mid-section. You defeat the purpose of trying to lose belly fat if you don't eat breakfast.

6. **Stir fry don't deep fry** — Often, people think they're "stir-frying," but use so much oil that they might as well be

deep frying their vegetables. Instead of using a lot of oil, just use a drop of oil to start. Then, gradually add water and let the vegetables stir-fry in their moisture. This not only reduces your fat intake but also makes the vegetables taste better.

7. **Heat your skillet when you fry** — If you take the time to heat your skillet before you add the oil, the oil gets hot quicker and less oil will be absorbed by your food. If you put oil in a cold skillet and add the meats or vegetables, the oil will soak into the food. If it soaks into the food, where does it go? It goes right into your body and adds belly fat.

8. **Camouflage your portions** — Sometimes, it isn't how much you eat that makes you full, it's how much you "think" you've eaten. When you have a flat small piece of meat on your plate it seems like you've been deprived. If you slice the meat thinly and stack it on your plate, it appears to be a bigger portion, so you think you've eaten more. This works for vegetables as well. A small potato sliced up will look larger. You'll think you're eating more than you are.

9. **Marinade without oil** — If you marinate in oil, the oil is soaked into the food, so naturally, it will be eaten. One recipe for the oil-free marinade is to combine apple juice (about 3 cups) pressed garlic (2 cloves) and soy sauce that is reduced to sodium (about 1 cup). Marinating healthily can greatly reduce the amount of fat you intake.

10. **Stuff food** — If you fill the centres of your food with wholesome ingredients, you'll be eating as much food, but reducing your caloric intake. Here are a few examples of this:

- Take your hamburger and scoop a hole in the middle of the meat before you cook it. Fill it with some type of vegetable such as mushrooms, olives, or whatever else you like. Then, if you've used the recommended serving size of three ounces, you've made it look much bigger, made it more filling, and made it much leaner. If you would have added more ounces of hamburger to make it that size, it would have been much less healthy.

- Stuff your meatballs with grated carrots, zucchini, or squash. This will add vitamins and moisture as well as size to your meatballs without changing the flavour. You'll be able to make your meatballs bigger, and not add calories and fat.

11. **Swap your food** — Sometimes, if you stop to think about it, you can think of substituting something healthier for something full of fat in your favourite recipes. By doing that, you'll be keeping that fat from settling in your mid-section and reducing that dreaded belly fat. Here are a few examples to get you started:

- When you make curry, use plain yoghurt instead of coconut milk which is full of fat. You'll get a good, creamy texture, but you won't have all the fat.

- Replace two slices of bread with one piece of pita bread — Folding a piece of pita bread will allow you to put more vegetables on your sandwich. More vegetables make it more filling, and you'll be making a much healthier sandwich.

- Replace red meat with lentils—In foods such as lasagna, only use about half the amount of ground beef. Add red lentils to make it filling. They're packed with protein, fat-free, and high in fibre. The flavour of red lentils is neutral, so they'll just absorb the flavour of your sauce and you won't notice the difference.

- **Substitute "turkey" versions of your favourite meat** —You can have turkey ham, turkey burger, turkey hot dogs, turkey bologna, or even turkey pepperoni. Turkey isn't nearly as high in fat as other meats. You'll have the flavour of the other meats without that added fat to carry around.

12. **Change the toppings on your pizza** — If you must have pepperoni on your pizza, consider adding at least two vegetable toppings. If you do this for every meat ordered as a topping, you'll have a healthier pizza. The carcinogens in meats that are processed have been found to increase your risk of cancer, so you'll not only be reducing your belly fat, you'll be improving your health.

13. **Use oats to stuff meat recipes** — Use oats that are in the same amount as other things you fill with such as crackers or bread crumbs. Not only are oats better for you, but because they have high fibre content, they taste the same, and can help you reduce your cholesterol.

14. **Use a healthier, low-fat recipe to replace your "fish-n-chips" recipe** — Use white fish such as cod or haddock and cut it into strips. Use sparkling water and self-rising flour for a light batter mix. Fry the strips in a small amount of canola oil. Instead of deep-fried French fries, cut potatoes and bake at 450 degrees in canola oil that you season with things like herbs, salt, garlic, etc.

15. **Reduce cheese in your toppings** — If you have a recipe that calls for a grated cheese topping, you can reduce fat and add fibre by replacing half of the cheese with whole-

wheat bread crumbs. The crumbs keep the texture of the baked cheese, so you won't know the difference.

16. **Eat healthier deli meats** — Deli meats aren't all bad, you just need to learn to eat the healthier ones. In order of health, the first would be chicken or turkey. The second is roast beef. The third is ham. Lastly, are all the other processed deli meats such as bologna, salami, olive loaf, etc.

17. **Don't drown your food** — You may or may not be old enough to remember Timer from the science portion of School House Rock watched in your Saturday morning cartoons. If you do, then you know he had a slogan: Don't drown your food in catsup or mayo or goo. It's no fun to eat what you can't even see, so don't drown your food! How many times have you seen someone prepare a nice, healthy salad only to pile on so much fattening dressing that it's no longer healthy? People will also pile on so much gravy that a lean piece of roast beef or turkey becomes unhealthy. Topping with meat natural juices instead or using extra virgin olive oil that is seasoned on salads will keep your food healthy and won't sacrifice the taste.

18. **Don't eat tuna salad with a lot of fattening mayonnaise** — Instead, you can add hot sauce, lemon juice, and pepper to your tuna. It tastes great and adds no fat.

19. **Use grated cheese instead of slices**—Grate hard cheeses such as Parmesan on your sandwiches. You'll get all the cheese flavour with much less fat.

20. **Have meals without meat**—I'm not saying go Vegan, but every meal doesn't have to be a "meat and potato" meal. Eat vegetarian lasagna and go without beef. Prepare eggplant parmesan instead of veal parmesan. You'll be taking in less fat, so there'll be less fat to stay around your middle.

21. **Use squash instead of a lot of cheese** — By adding pureed butternut squash to half the cheese mixture in foods like macaroni and cheese, quesadillas, or grilled sandwiches will reduce the calorie count without altering the taste of the food. Squash is high in vitamins and potassium, so not only will your food have less fat and calories, it will be healthier.

22. **Use greens to wrap your meat**—Instead of eating meats that are between two slices of bread, wrap them in a large lettuce leaf or some other leafy green such as romaine lettuce, or Chinese cabbage. You'll be reducing your intake of carbohydrates that can add belly fat.

23. **Use avocados instead of mayonnaise** — Ripe avocados will make your sandwich moist like mayonnaise, and have good fat instead of bad fat. This can also lower your cholesterol.

24. **Make your pancakes healthier** — Cornmeal is healthier than traditional flour. It has higher fibre content, as well as magnesium. For healthier pancakes, replace half your flour with cornmeal. They'll have a great texture and be better for you.

25. **Make sure you get all the vitamins from your cereal** —If you've taken the steps to eat healthier breakfast cereals, you probably aren't getting all the nutrition from it that you should. To do so, you need to drink the milk in the bowl. As much as 40 per cent of the nutritional vitamins from your cereal will dissolve into the milk, so drinking it makes it healthier for you.

26. **Keep frozen bananas on hand** — Frozen bananas are great for making smoothies that are healthy and nutritious. They're sweet, so they eliminate the need for sugary ingredients. Frozen, they have the cold state for good thick smoothies and won't go bad quickly like they

can if they're unfrozen.

27. **Eat chocolate** — Yes, you read correctly. So often, people ignore their cravings for chocolate because they feel it is "bad" for them. Dark chocolate, however, is lower in fat and very high in antioxidants, so eating it will both satisfy your cravings and give you a healthy snack. You can also shave dark chocolate into dishes like barbecue sauce or chilli. It gives it a good flavour boost and will help you prevent heart disease as well as keep your cholesterol at a good level. If you want a good night-time snack, take two tablespoons of dark chocolate and melt it in the microwave. Stir it with 4 ounces of vanilla yoghurt and top it with about a tablespoon of almond slivers.

28. **Make your dips yourself** — Store-bought dips can be very high in fat content and calories. If you prepare your dips yourself, however, you can greatly reduce the fat and calories. Just use fat-free sour cream or yoghurt. You can mix it with an equal portion of salsa or add herbs and/or lemon. Whatever flavour you choose will be much healthier for you this way.

29. **Purchase nuts that are in shells** — If you have to spend time shelling the nuts, you'll spend less time eating big handfuls of them. Nuts in and of themselves can be healthy, especially pistachios, almonds and walnuts. If, however, you eat too many, they become like any other food you overeat and will cause you to gain weight.

30. **Boil your peanuts** — If you boil peanuts for a few hours, they will have approximately four times the amount of antioxidants they have prepared any other way. Boiled peanuts are a popular snack already in Asia, China, Australia, and the southern portion of the US. If you haven't tried them, the next time you want peanuts, give them a try.

31. **Balance your baked potatoes** — Many people give up baked potatoes because of their high glycemic rating. You can have them, however, if you balance them with a healthy topping like cheddar cheese, broccoli, mushrooms, or spinach.

32. **Rinse canned beans** — Beans such as kidney beans are a great way to add both fibre and protein to a meal. Canned beans, however, contain a lot of sodium. This can give you a bloated feeling as well as cause high blood pressure. Rinsing them, however, washes away that high sodium content and makes them healthy again.

33. **Make your side dishes thicker** — If you use evaporated milk that is fat-free in dishes like mashed potatoes or macaroni and cheese, you will give them a thicker texture that will seem more filling. In addition to that, you'll be taking in more calcium per cup without all the fat.

34. **Serve yourself water as an appetizer** — Water is filling, cleansing, and keeps you properly hydrated. If you drink two glasses of water before each meal, you will fill up quickly and eat less.

35. **Add spice to your life** — Research has found that people that were overweight will become slimmer if they eat meals that contain Chile peppers. They contain capsaicin. It's what makes them hot, and it helps the liver clear insulin from your bloodstream after you eat. Since insulin is the hormone that tells your body to store the fat, clearing it from the body can reduce belly fat.

36. **Avoid emotional eating** — Sometimes people use food as a comfort. When you're hurt or upset, you turn to food to make you feel better. When you feel like eating just to eat and you know you're not hungry, substitute it with something else like going on a bike. If you must eat

something, make it fresh fruits or vegetables.

While exercise is an essential part of weight loss, you should realize that exercises that target your abdominal area won't help you burn the fat. They will define the muscles there, but to achieve those abs, you first have to get rid of all the fat you have in your belly. Here are a few tips you can use to exercise your way to less belly fat:

37. **Walk** — Try to get in at least 10,000 steps every day. If you have a sedentary job, this may be difficult for you. Schedule a time and place to do brisk walking every day. If you can't, then choose a few other walking activities like parking at the far end of the parking lot at work or when you go to grocery or department stores. Take the steps instead of the elevator.

38. **Aerobic exercise or aerobic dancing** — Aerobics are a great way to get a good cardio workout. You can do this in a group, such as a class, or get an exercise video and do them in the privacy of your own home. Whichever way you choose, getting up your cardio rate will help your body burn fat. The exercise or dancing part of aerobic exercise will help reduce fat and build muscle.

39. **Ride a bike** — Biking, when done at a cardio pace, is a great way to get a good workout and burn calories. Many people who don't have the time in their busy days to do a workout get their exercise from biking to and from work each day. You can jump-start your metabolism each morning with a good ride, and then reduce the stress of a hectic day on the ride home.

40. **Jog** — Jogging isn't for everyone, but many people stay fit and trim from jogging. You can do this outdoors, on an indoor track, or a treadmill. If you're over 50, you want to check with your physician to be sure you're physically fit for jogging. Many times the jar from jogging on the knees,

hips, and/or back can be harmful to those with problems. Once you've got a clean bill of health, "Run Forest, Run!"

41. **Take a martial arts class** — Martial arts classes are good for cardio workouts, muscle definition, and self-defence. They can also be a lot of fun. If you're hesitant to join a class alone, talk a friend into joining you.

42. **Weight training or Pilates** — Either of these, in conjunction with a good cardio workout, can help you build muscle. Muscles will burn calories. You can find free weight training workouts for beginners to advanced, and Pilates classes are available for all levels as well. Cardio three to five times a week with a good weight training program will help you burn overall body fat, and that includes that dreaded belly fat.

43. **Breath control exercises** — Another supplemental exercise is breath control exercises that are good for the abdominal region. Yoga is a prime example. Though it is optional, and not essential for reducing belly fat, it is a simple way to strengthen the abdominal area and remove inches from your waistline.

44. **Keep good posture** — Although you might not realize it, you use many core muscles simply to hold yourself up straight in good posture. Keeping good posture while tightening your stomach muscles can strengthen both the back muscles and the abdominal muscles.

45. **Simple leg lifts** —To tighten the abdominal muscles, lay flat on your back. Raise your feet about two inches off the ground and hold them to a slow count of ten. Lower your feet and then do it again. Try to do this at least 10 times a day. It is a simple basic way to begin to strengthen weakened abdominal muscles.

46. **Try exercising in small bursts** — Research shows that alternating bursts of energy, just small ones, with brief

resting periods can not only improve your muscle tone and burn calories but can also build endurance. This is a good way to get started and build up to the more serious exercises. You might try sprinting. Just run as fast as you can for around 20 seconds. Walk until your breathing returns to normal, and do it again. If you do this for about 10 minutes a day, you'll be on your way to a good start.

Set your exercise equipment for interval training—In this mode, it increases the difficulty for short periods and then returns to normal. It gives you the effect of exercising in small bursts by using machines.

47. **Snack first** — If you're going out for a business dinner or to a party of some kind, eat a healthy, high-protein snack before you go. This will make you less hungry and will allow you to eat smaller portions of the more fattening foods.

48. **Fit some type of exercise into your normal work day** —This can be difficult for some people. It all depends on the type of job you have. You might set aside your lunch hours for walking. If that's not possible, plan five minutes out of each day for a power walk. Take long, brisk strides when you walk down the hall or go up and down stairs.

49. **Stretch the sides of your waist** — With one arm over your head, lean as far as you can to the opposite side. Then switch hands. This will strengthen the muscles of your waistline. It will tone them, and remember muscle burns fat, so having good muscle tone is important.

50. When all else fails, there's always surgery—If you've tried everything and you just can't get rid of your belly fat, there are two types of surgery you could consider.

- Tummy tuck—This is also referred to as an abdominoplasty. It takes out the excessive fat and skin you have stored in your midsection. It can usually reestablish weakened muscles which gives you a firmer abdominal area.

- Panniculectomy—This can be done by itself or along with an abdominoplasty. It removes any overhanging skin and tissue known as an "apron" from below the naval. This skin usually occurs when people have had excessive weight loss.

If you have overhanging skin, it can cause you a lot of problems. It would pull on your back, causing back pain. It can also cause hygiene problems and yeast infections. Sometimes cysts develop in the folds. If you have this overhanging skin, it shouldn't be ignored.

Conclusion

Though people may be happy with their inner selves and with who they are as a person, not many people will say they're happy about being overweight. If you're unhappy with yourselves, it's time to get motivated to lose weight. If you want to lose weight and keep it off, you'll need a lot of motivation. It isn't just about going on a diet. It's a complete, total lifestyle change. You've had the habit of overeating for a long time. It takes time to get rid of those habits and establish new ones. Once you've established the new ones, however, you can begin shedding that belly fat.

Remember, losing weight is only half the battle. Keeping the weight off can often be harder than losing it. If you want to keep it off, you have to commit to a lifestyle change. If you go back to your old habits, you can gain all the weight you lost and more. You have to find new eating habits that you can live with. They have to be habits you can sustain for a lifetime.

Make sure you keep your regimen of healthy eating and exercise. Even if you opt for tip 50 and have surgery, the weight can still return.

If motivation is difficult for you, find someone who can give you support and encourage you. It may be your doctor, your spouse, a friend or another family member. This often helps you stay on track.

Sometimes it's hard to make lifestyle changes that suit us. They need to go along with our physical fitness and overall state of health. You want to be sure to talk to your doctor. He/she can help you weigh all the options and decide what plan of action works best for you. Your goal is to have long-term success. You may have to try different options to find out what works for you.

Sometimes, in your weight-loss process, you may get stuck. You lose a certain amount of weight and just can't lose any more. It's important not to give up. You've set a weight-loss goal, and you want to reach it. To do so, sometimes all you have to do is make a few minor changes to what you're doing. You can reduce your calories a bit or increase your exercise. Walk the extra mile. Whatever you can find that gives you that push over the edge and jump-starts you again. Whatever you do, don't give up. You'll get excited about seeing your waistline reduce and be motivated to press on. If you get stuck, however, it can be a bit disheartening.

Sometimes, you may be motivated by health improvements. You can check your cholesterol levels. If they decrease, you know you're reducing your chances of heart disease. You may see regular blood pressure for the first time in years. Your breathing may improve and you'll be able to do a lot more than you used to. These things are motivators to keep the weight off many people. If you're losing weight for health reasons, however, note that sometimes it takes a while for these interventions to kick in.

You didn't become unhealthy overnight, and losing a few pounds isn't going to instantly change that. It is a gradual process, so keep pressing forward. Eventually, you'll see the results.

It is important to remember that you may not be able to lose weight the way your Great Aunt Ruth did. You may go on a diet with a friend and they may lose and you may not. Remember that you didn't gain the weight at the same rate or by eating and doing the same thing. All bodies are different. They work in different ways. What works for you might not work for your friends either. You have to find something that works for YOU! Don't stop until you've found something. Get to know your own body and how it works. That will help you find the right solution and combination of foods and exercises that work best for you.

Know that doing 100 crunches a day for the rest of your life won't reduce your belly fat. Too many people believe that and are greatly disappointed when they work that hard and have nothing to show for it. You have to reduce your intake of processed carbohydrates and eat fat-burning proteins instead.

For unknown reasons, belly fat just seems to burn slower than the fat on the rest of your body. You didn't get that belly overnight, and you won't lose it overnight either. The good news is, however, that it does burn! It may take a few weeks to see progress, but keep it up and you will see it.

It isn't easy to lose weight and then keep it off. If you've accomplished this, it is an important achievement. You probably feel good about yourself, but don't be surprised if you find that you are better able to face other challenges and also succeed in them. Sometimes eating healthier is easier than exercising. One good tip to keep exercising is if you're having a bad day and you don't feel like exercising, go halfway. Get in your car and go to the gym. Once you get there, you might not want to go in. That's fine. At least driving yourself there is a step. Usually, you'll think, "Well, I'm here, I might as well go in." Once you do, those endorphins kick in and you find yourself enjoying the exercise and greatly benefiting from it.

As you go along, you can measure your progress using what is known as your "waist-to-hip" ratio. To do this, you measure the narrowest part of your waist and the broadest portion of your hips. Then you divide the circumference of your waistline by the circumference of your hips. Just divide the waist measurement by the hip measurement. A woman should have a ratio that is 0.8 or lower. A man should have a ratio of 0.9 or lower.

Don't rely on your memory. Write down your progress. Keep all your measurements written down together in some place so you can easily chart your progress as you go. This can be a big encouragement and motivator to keep going. When you're measuring, make sure you weigh yourself at the same time of the day each time. Weight can fluctuate during different parts of the day. This can be predicted by your last meal or your last bowel movement. By measuring at the same time of the day, you'll get a better idea of your true weight loss. Most people find the morning before breakfast as the best time.

When you feel yourself having difficulty being motivated to exercise, try putting forth half of the effort. At least get in your car and go over to the gym. You can always turn around and go home if you don't feel like it once you get there. Chances are, however, you'll feel, "I've made it this far, I might as well go in and give exercising a try." Don't commit to a full exercise routine. Just commit to working on the bicycle for 10 minutes. Once you do that, you can commit to one more thing at a time until you finish. If, however, you don't feel like it, at least you can say you tried. Once those endorphins kick in, however, you'll probably feel like it. You'll probably feel much better when you're finished.

If you're tired of belly fat and desperate to lose weight, don't take those desperate measures some people take. They starve themselves, try every fad diet that comes out, or take expensive supplements that don't work just because they all say you will lose weight immediately. Losing that belly fat just isn't going to happen overnight. Yo-yo dieting will only mess up your body's metabolism and cause you to gain more weight than you lost in the first place. Starving causes you to binge at the first temptation of something you love to eat. Your system gets so confused, it's no wonder that belly fat stays.

Keeping your body's metabolism running effectively and continuously burning calories is what will help you prevent that fat storage around your midsection and keep you from gaining weight again. When you eat healthy foods and exercise you'll develop lean muscle mass which will allow you to intake calories and not gain weight because muscle helps burn fat.

Don't forget as you begin the weight-loss process, you need to set realistic goals. If your goals aren't realistic and achievable, then you'll become discouraged. You'll lose confidence in yourself and give up easier. Setting realistic goals will help give you that boost of confidence each time you reach one to move forward in your weight loss.

9 798889 592174

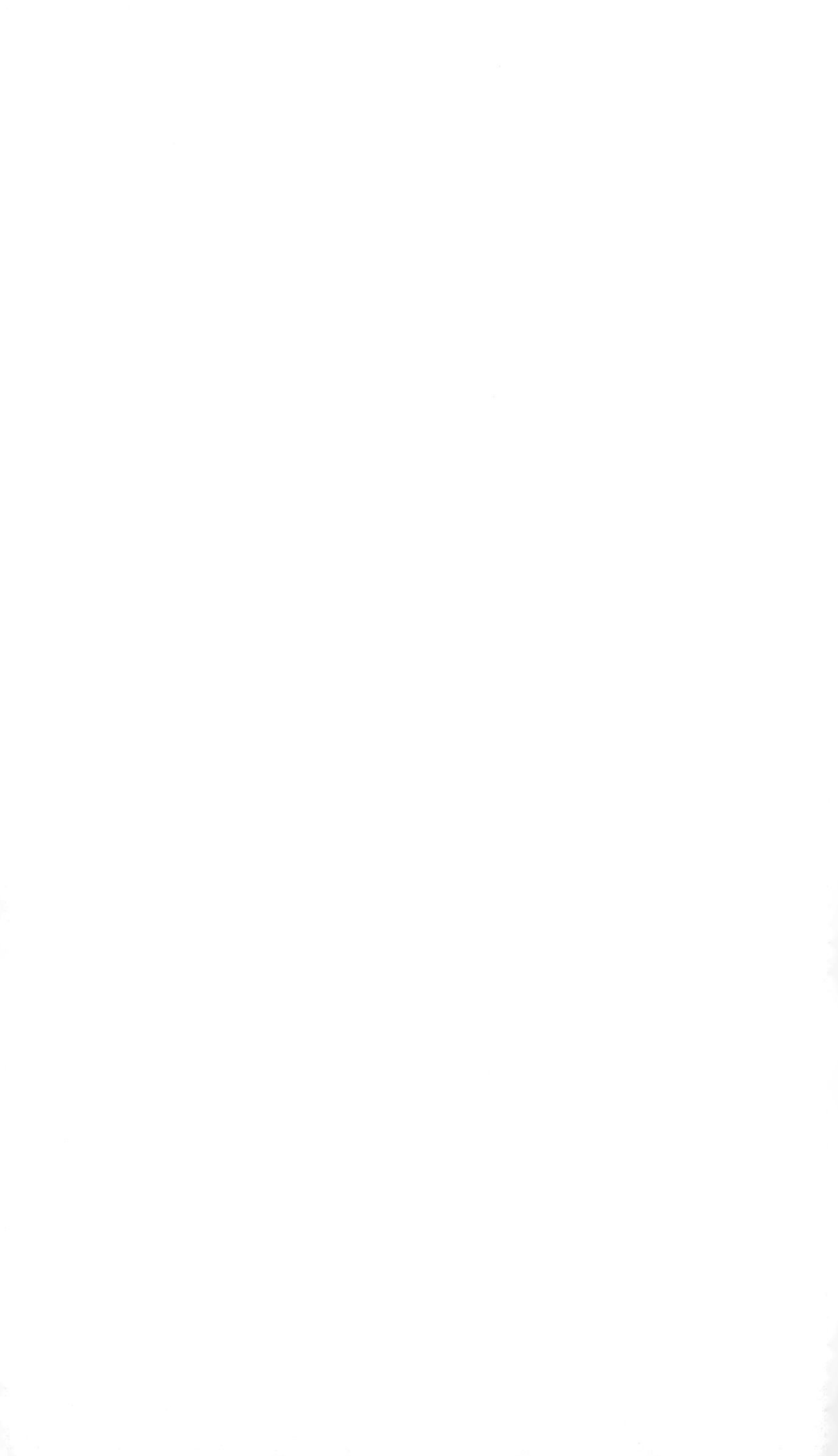

Printed by Libri Plureos GmbH in Hamburg,
Germany